Paleo Mexican Recipes

Preparing the Simple Tex-Mex Paleo Cuisines At Home

I0438882

Disclaimer

The author has tried to be an authentic source of the information provided in this report. However, the author does not oppose the additional information available over the internet. The objective of providing different Mexican recipes is to enable readers to try these delicious recipes at home. The recipes included in this book cannot be compared with the preparation methods of the same provided in other books. All readers can seek further help through additional sources of information. Also, the pictures in the book may appear different from the actual recipe.

Ignoring any of the guidelines or not following each step of the preparation method of Mexican dishes may not give you the exact result. Therefore, the author is not responsible for such negligence.

Summary

It is very common to desire an array of flavors on our dining table on a daily basis. With a wide variety of specialties from around the world, our wish to enjoy different types of food is pretty justified.

Tangy Sichuan scorchers and pad Thai, intricate curries from India, Japanese special sushi, Vietnamese herby-fresh spring-rolls and authentic Italian squash pasta with chili and garlic and of course, lots of spicy Mexican food!

Talk about Mexican cuisine and the first few dishes you can recall are the Mexican-American burritos and tacos served with sour cream and salsa or Mexican squash pasta infused with cilantro and jalapenos. These are some common Mexican dishes we enjoy regularly. However, talk about real Mexican cuisine and the options are endless.

Mexican food is in the options for you even if you follow Paleo diet. If you haven't tried a full range of Paleo Mexican menu on your dining table yet, this is your chance. This book has the widest range of most exotic, versatile and authentic Paleo Mexican recipes to prepare the best Mexican food at home.

What will you find in this book?

- ➢ Most authentic 50 Paleo Mexican recipes
- ➢ Easy to prepare recipes
- ➢ Exotically flavorful and pure Mexican taste
- ➢ Easy to find Ingredients
- ➢ Each recipe with nutritional information
- ➢ Divided into 8 different categories

So if you are ready to experience the real Mexican taste without cheating on your diet, try the recipes shared in this book and have an amazing dining time with friends and family.

Contents

Mexican Appetizers: Savory Sidelines and Starters

Indeed, no Mexican dish is complete without an interesting sideline or starter. Mexican food is known for its peppery range of flavors, which are combined together to make a dish worth relishing.

Check out these interesting appetizers below and match with your favorite main course from the list to enjoy the perfect Paleo Mexican dining experience.

Note: Nutritional facts for each recipe are given on a single serving basis.

Paleo-Friendly Mexican Tortillas

Before we jump to the recipes, check out the perfect Paleo tortillas recipe below. Tortillas are essential for most Mexican recipe. Use this recipe to prepare Paleo-friendly tortillas with all the recipes you want.

Ingredients

2 large eggs, whisked
Olive oil, 1 tbsp
Almond milk (unsweetened), 1 cup
Tapioca flour, ¾ cup
Coconut flour (sifted), 3 tbsp
Sea salt, ¼ tsp

Preparation Method

In a bowl, add almond milk, whisked eggs and olive oil and mix together.

In another bowl, add all the dry ingredients including tapioca flour, coconut flour and sea sold and toss to combine.

Now add the wet mixture to the dry mixture and whisk to fully combine.

To cook, heat oil in a non-stick pan. Pour ⅓ cup batter into the center and with the help of a large spoon form a circle spreading the batter. Make around 6" circle.

Let it cook untouched for 2-3 minutes over low-med heat until tortilla is browned on the bottom. Flip to cook the other side for a few minutes. When done, remove from the pan and place tortillas on paper towel-lined serving plate. Prepare more with the remaining batter.

You can slice these tortillas into small triangles and serve with any Mexican recipe you like. Enjoy the delicious recipes below:

Chicken Tortilla Soup

Serves 8

With a range of interesting, Mexican-special ingredients, prepare a relishing soup that will be a perfect starter for an authentic Mexican menu. The combination of flavors used will create a magical taste that will serve your taste buds just the right way.

Total Time Required

1 hour 10 minutes

Nutritional Facts

Calories: 398
Cholesterol: 74mg
Carbohydrates: 28g
Protein: 29g
Fat: 19g

Ingredients

Carrot (diced), 1 cup
Celery, 1cup
Onion (diced), 1 cup
Garlic powder, ½ tsp or fresh garlic (diced), ½ tsp
Sea salt, ⅛ tsp
Pepper, ¼ tsp
Almond oil, 1 tbsp
Chicken Broth, 4 cans or 15oz.
Tomatoes (diced), 1 can of 15 oz (optional)
Chilies (diced), ½ tbsp
Jalapenos (diced and deseeded), ½ tbsp
Taco seasoning, 1 packet (Paleo friendly)
10 tortillas (8"), cut into small 1" pieces (choose Paleo-friendly version)
Chicken meat (poached and diced), 12 oz.
Homemade dairy-free sour cream, 1 cup
grass-fed grass fed cheese (shredded), 12 oz

Preparation Method

To prepare dairy-free sour cream, place 1 can of coconut milk in the refrigerator for at least 4 hours or overnight for best results. The cream will separate from the milk. Open the can and scrape out the cream only and place it in a small bowl. Add sea salt and 2 tbsp lemon juice and whisk until well combined. Add more salt or lemon juice if required. Your sour cream is now ready to be used.

Place skillet over low-med flame and heat oil. Add onions and carrots and sauté. Sprinkle salt and pepper, mix and cook until tender.

Stir in chicken broth next and bring the mixture to boil.

Add tomatoes, chilies, jalapenos, chicken and taco seasoning to the skillet. Mix to combine.

Add small pieces of tortilla into the broth mixture and stir. Let the mixture boil for 20-22 minutes until tortillas are nicely blended into the soup. Stir occasionally to keep the soup from sticking.

Reduce the flame to low and add grass fed cheese (8 oz. only). Mix and let it simmer for 8-10 minutes. Add sour cream and simmer the soup for another 10 minutes.

To adjust the consistency of the soup and to make it thicker, you can add more tortillas in the soup and let it incorporate in the mixture. When done, turn the stove off and pour the soup in a large serving bowl.

Garnish with crushed tortilla chips and remaining grass fed cheese. Serve hot and enjoy.

Classic Tex-Mex Guacamole

Serves 4

An authentic Mexican menu is incomplete without a classic, all-time-favorite Guacamole. With basic ingredients and a little flavorful twist, this sideline will surely complete your full Mexican meal. A must-have sideline for pure Tex-Mex dining experience!

Total Time Required

1 hour 10 minutes

Nutritional Facts

Calories: 154
Cholesterol: 3mg
Carbohydrates: 8.5g
Protein: 2g
Fat: 14g

Ingredients

6 Avocados (ripe)
Juice of 3 limes
1 medium-sized yellow onion (chopped)
Fresh garlic (minced), 1 clove
2 Serrano chilies (cut into circles)
Fresh cilantro (stems intact, chopped finely), ½ cup
Olive oil, ¼ tsp
Sea salt, to taste
Pepper, to taste

Preparation Method

Slice the avocados into halves and pit. Scoop out the avocados flesh with the help of a spoon into a mixing bowl. Mash it with a potato masher or fork, leaving it a little chunky. Stir in the remaining ingredients including lime juice, chopped onion, garlic, Serrano chilies and cilantro. Mix well.

Add seasoning with pepper and salt and drizzle the mixture with olive oil. Give all the ingredients a thorough mix with a fork.

Now cover the bowl with a plastic wrap nicely to keep it fresh and refrigerate guacamole for at least 60 minutes. Serve chilled with tortilla chips or any other Mexican dish you like.

Lime Soup

Lime Soup
Serves 4

Orzo and Lime Soup is a perfect, savory starter for a delicious Mexican menu. The distinctive ingredients make the flavor very unique. The soup is prepared with a combination of squash pasta, veggies, jalapeno, chicken cilantro, and of course lime juice!

Total Time Required

45 minutes

Nutritional Facts

Calories: 338
Cholesterol: 54.4mg
Carbohydrates: 34.7g
Protein: 29.3g
Fat: 9.7g

Ingredients

Olive oil, 1 ½ tbsp
1 medium-sized white onion (thinly sized)
Garlic (thinly sliced), 6 cloves
2 jalapenos (thinly sliced)
Chicken breast (skinless, boneless), ¾ lb cut into very thin and small strips
Chicken broth (low sodium), 5 cup
Fresh lime juice, ¼ cup
Fresh cilantro (chopped), ¼ cup
1 large-sized tomato (seeded and chopped)
Fresh cilantro, for garnish
Sea salt, ¼ tsp
Pepper, ¼ tsp

Preparation Method

Set a large saucepan over low-med heat and add oil. When the oil is little warm, stir in onion, chilies and garlic. Sauté the ingredients until onion changes color to light brown for about 2-4 minutes.

Add chicken in the saucepan and cook for another minute. Add tomato, lime juice and broth next and stir well. Simmer your soup for about 3-4 minutes until chicken is properly cooked.

Add chopped cilantro.

Sprinkle salt and pepper and mix. Turn off the stove and ladle the soup in a large serving bowl. Garnish with cilantro and enjoy hot.

Fried Grass fed cheese
Serves 2

Prepared with only three ingredients, this Tex-Mex specialty can enhance the flavors of any food. Add it as a sideline or serve it as a starter, Mexican-style fried grass fed cheese is a must-have on a Mexican dining table.

Total Time Required

5 minutes

Nutritional Facts

Calories: 310
Cholesterol: 30mg
Carbohydrates: 23g
Protein: 10g
Fat: 19g

Ingredients

Panela or Queso blanco grass fed cheese, 1 block
Olive oil, ½ cup
Garlic powder, ½ tsp

Preparation Method

Cut grass fed cheese into small cubes about 1"- 2" in size. In a small frying pan, heat oil over med-high heat. Carefully add the grass fed cheese cubes in the oil. Let cook for a few seconds on one side and then flip using a spoon. Cook on each side for a few seconds until it's done from all sides.

When done, remove and place it on a plate with paper towel to drain oil. Sprinkle garlic powder on the top to enjoy friend grass fed cheese with garlic bread flavor.

Can add to any dish as a sideline.

Mexican Dips – The Perfect Mexican Flavor

Mexican Dips are essential part of an authentic Mexican dining experience. Make any homemade dish a champion-winning recipe by adding an interesting dip mentioned below.

The recipes we have compiled for you here are very versatile with different ingredients and flavors to give you a unique experience every time.

Simple to make, nutritionally rich and very interesting! Check out yourself.

Chili-Grass fed cheese Dip

Serves 2-3

One of the most filling and spicy grass fed cheese dip can now be made at home with absolutely authentic Paleo ingredients. Takes only a few minutes to prepare and can be served with Paleo-Friendly tortillas or any other Mexican dish you like.

Total Time Required

10-12 minutes

Nutritional Facts

Calories: 104.4
Cholesterol: 7.3mg
Carbohydrates: 8.6g
Protein: 12g
Fat: 2.3g

Ingredients

Grass-fed grass fed cheese, 2 cups
Almond milk, ½ cup
Chili powder, 1 tsp
Fresh tomatoes (diced). ⅓ cup
Green onion (sliced), ⅓ cup
Canned green chilies (mild flavor), ¼ cup
Cilantro sprig (optional)
1 small chili pepper (optional)

Preparation Method

Set a saucepan over low-med heat. Add grass fed cheese, milk, chili powder and combine. Cook for around 6-8 minutes, stirring constantly, to melt grass fed cheese and combine all ingredients well.

Turn off the stove, stir in diced tomatoes, chilies and green onion. Pour into a serving bowl. Garnish with cilantro and chili pepper if desired.

Mexican Nacho Dip
Serves 2-3

Stop turning your head away from the most delicious Mexican Nacho Dip. With amazing alternative ingredients, you can now make warm and delectable nacho dip at home – absolutely Paleo. Serve with Paleo Nachos and enjoy!

Total Time Required

10-12 minutes

Nutritional Facts

Calories: 113
Cholesterol: 6.6mg
Carbohydrates: 8g
Protein: 1.3g
Fat: 12g

Ingredients

Cashews (soaked in water for 4 hours-12 hours), 1 cup
Coconut water, 6 tbsp
Grass-fed goat grass fed cheese, ¼ cup
Olive oil, 1 tbsp
1 jalapeno (chopped)
Paprika, ½ tsp
Chili powder, 1 tsp
Sea salt, to taste
Garlic salt, to taste
Onion powder, to taste
Serrano chilies, a few

Preparation Method

Combine all ingredients in a blender and blend for 6-8 minutes at different speed levels to make a thick, creamy dip. You can adjust the consistency by adding more grass fed cheese or coconut water.

Adjust the taste by adding as many chilies as you want. Just make it your own!

Pour out the mixture in a small serving bowl. Heat it for a minute in a microwave before serving. Tastes delicious with Paleo nachos!

Zesty Tomato-Garlic Dip
Serves 12 (2 tbsp each)

Enjoy the delicious blend of tomatoes and garlic and experience fresh-flavored dip with your favorite Mexican recipe at any hour of the day. You can even serve with Paleo-friendly tortillas and enjoy the flavors to the fullest.

Total Time Required

10 minutes

Nutritional Facts

Calories: 98
Cholesterol: 12.1mg
Carbohydrates: 1.5g
Protein: 0.5g
Fat: 10g

Ingredients

Tomatoes (sun-dried), 1 cup
Mayonnaise (dairy-free), ¾ cup
Garlic (minced), 3 tbsp
Grass-fed goat grass fed cheese (grated), 2 tbsp
Lemon juice, ½ tbsp
Onion powder, ½ tsp
Black pepper, ¼ tsp
Garlic salt, ¼ tsp
Fresh parsley, few sprigs

Preparation Method

Add mayonnaise, garlic, tomatoes, grass fed cheese, onion powder, lemon juice, pepper, parsley and garlic salt in a blender. Pulse the blender at high until the ingredients make a thick, creamy blend. Garnish with parsley.

Enjoy the dip with your favorite corn-free tortillas. Warm the dip in a microwave before eating if you like.

Roasted Cashew-Tomato Mexican Dip

Serves 2 cups

This roasted dip made of tomato and cashews is definitely a very unique combination to serve your taste buds. With pure Mexican flavors and ingredients, enjoy the Paleo version with absolutely no compromise in the taste.

Total Time Required

30 minutes

Nutritional Facts

Calories: 159
Cholesterol: 13.5mg
Carbohydrates: 5.3g
Protein: 1.5g
Fat: 36g

Ingredients

4 tomatoes (quartered)
Garlic, 2 cloves
Olive oil, 2 tbsp (divided)
Raw honey, ½ tbsp
Sea salt, to taste
Ground black pepper, to taste
Cashews, 1 cup (soaked in water for 3-6 hours)
Tahini, 1 tbsp
Basil leaves, ½ cup
Balsamic vinegar, ½ tbsp

Preparation Method

Set the oven to preheat at 400°F. Prepare and great a baking sheet and set aside.

In a large bowl, toss together tomatoes, honey, olive oil (1 tbsp), salt and pepper. Spread the mixture on the baking sheet.

Chop off garlic clove tips, drizzle in remaining olive oil and use an aluminum foil to wrap it. Place it on the baking sheet.

Set to bake for 20-25 minutes. When done, remove and place on a cooling rack and allow to cool for 5-10 minutes.

Meanwhile, grind cashews in a blender or food processer until smooth, for around 2 minutes.

Add in the remaining ingredients, including tomato mixture and garlic in the processor and pulse again. Blend until all ingredients are fully incorporated. Make sure you scrape the sides as well.

Serve in a serving bowl and season with additional pepper and salt. Enjoy!

Mexican Salsa – Sweet and Sour Salsa

Nothing can be compared with the fountain of flavors offered by Mexican salsa. It is hard to believe that such flavorful recipes can be made in a pure Paleo version.

However, the following recipes will make your dream of eating authentic Paleo Mexican Salsa come true! Try them yourself.

Refreshing Tomato Salsa
Serves 2 cups

Tomatoes, salt and lots of lime juice are the best part of this salsa recipe. Without skimping on the hot chilies, prepare a salsa recipe with ripe, fresh tomatoes. Tomatoes without the burst of heat in this recipe are simply chopped tomatoes. So add flavors and enjoy!

Total Time Required

5 minutes

Nutritional Facts

Calories: 120
Cholesterol: 30mg
Carbohydrates: 2.5g
Protein: 8g
Fat: 9g

Ingredients

Tomatoes (seeded and diced), ¾ lb
Cilantro (chopped), ⅓ cup
White onion (finely chopped), ¼ cup
Jalapeno or Serrano chilies (finely chopped, with seeds), according to taste
Lime juice (freshly squeezed), 1 tbsp
Sea salt, 1 tsp

Preparation Method

Place all ingredients in a bowl. Toss to combine. Season with salt, lime juice and jalapeno pepper or Serrano chili. Adjust flavors according to your required taste.

Garlic-Tomatillo Salsa
Serves 2 cups

Tomatillos along with hot jalapenos and garlic give this delicious salsa a very earthy, rich flavor. Don't hesitate in adding roasted Jamaican scotch bonnets to the recipe if you like your salsa very hot and peppery.

Total Time Required

40 minutes

Nutritional Facts

Calories: 50
Cholesterol: 0mg
Carbohydrates: 10g
Protein: 0g
Fat: 0g

Ingredients

Fresh tomatillos (without husks), 1 lb
1 head garlic (peeled and separated)
3-4 Jalapeno peppers
Water, ½ cup
Fresh cilantro, 1 bunch
Sea salt, to taste
Ground black pepper, to taste

Ingredients

Set the oven broiler to preheat.

Arrange garlic cloves, jalapenos and tomatillos evenly on a baking sheet. Set to cook under the broiler for a few minutes. When toasted, remove garlic first. Let tomatillos and jalapenos to roast a little more, until they are evenly charred. Turn the sides as you cook.

When done, remove from the oven and place it on a cooling rack. Let the ingredients cool completely. Do not remove charred parts of pepper or tomatillos. They will give your salsa a very nice, deep flavor.

Now add tomatillos, peppers, cilantro and garlic in a blender. Add water and blend to prepare a thick, smooth mixture. Pour in a serving bowl and season with salt, pepper and lime juice (optional). Set your delicious tomatillo salsa in the refrigerator for 30-40 minutes before serving. Enjoy chilled.

Fruity Mango Salsa

Serves 1 cup

Enjoy the refreshing, fruity salsa recipe with sweet flavors of mango and sour flavors of lime juice and tomato salsa. The combination is mouth-watering and will enhance the taste of any dish you serve along!

Total Time Required

10 minutes

Nutritional Facts

Calories: 80
Cholesterol: 0mg
Carbohydrates: 16g
Protein: 0g
Fat: 0g

Ingredients

Tomato salsa (use recipe shared above), ¾ cup
1 large mango (ripe), peel and dice
Fresh cilantro (chopped), 2 tbsp
Lime juice (freshly squeezed), 2 tbsp

Preparation Method

In a serving bowl, add tomato salsa (you can prepare using the recipe above or can get a prepared paleo version from a superstore) along with mango, cilantro and lime juice.

Toss to incorporate flavors together. Tastes amazing with fish recipes!

Avocado Salsa
Serves 6

Total Time Required

10 minutes

Nutritional Facts

Calories: 107.4
Cholesterol: 0mg
Carbohydrates: 8.4g
Protein: 1.7g
Fat: 8.5g

Ingredients

2 medium-sized avocados (ripe), halved, pitted and peeled
2 vine-ripped tomatoes, (chopped and seeded)
1 red onion, (finely chopped), soak in ice water for 30 minutes and drain
1-2 jalapeno pepper (minced)
Fresh lime juice, 2 tbsp
Fresh cilantro leaves, 2 tbsp
Sea salt, to taste
Ground black pepper, 2 taste

Preparation Method

Chop peeled avocados and place them in a bowl. Add remaining ingredients one by one and stir to combine.

Season with salt and pepper and toss to combine flavors. Serve!

Note: You can prepare the salsa around 4 hours early. Cover with plastic and set to refrigerate. This will allow the flavors to settle more. Best serve at room temperature.

Watermelon Salsa
Serves 8

Watermelon and jalapenos – what a combination! The refreshing watermelon when combined with hot, peppery jalapenos will turn your meal more enjoyable and delicious. Add this salsa as a sideline or serve it as an appetizer with Paleo-friendly tortilla chips and enjoy!

Total Time Required

15 minutes

Nutritional Facts

Calories: 23
Cholesterol: 0mg
Carbohydrates: 6g
Protein: 1g
Fat: 8.5g

Ingredients

Watermelon (seedless, finely diced), 3 cups
2-3 jalapenos (seedless and minced)
Fresh cilantro (chopped), ⅓ cup
Red onion (minced), ¼ cup
Lime juice,3 tbsp
Sea salt, to taste
Paleo-friendly tortilla chips (to serve)

Preparation Method

In a glass bowl, add all the ingredients and toss to combine. Season with salt and toss again. Serve at room temperature or chilled (as you like). Accompany with tortilla chips and enjoy!

Mexican Breakfast: Your Morning Delight

Here's comes the turn of the most important meal of the day. Time to make the perfect Paleo Mexican breakfast!

So finally you will be making some real recipes that you can enjoy as your breakfast. These recipes below are made from Paleo ingredients so that you can enjoy the most delicious and healthy breakfast without cheating on your diet.

Ready to prepare your breakfast the Mexican way? Get started!

Egg Chilaquiles
Serves 2-4

Tired of partying all night? That's the perfect time to serve yourself with a delicious Mexican breakfast. This classic casserole recipe is a perfect dish to use your leftover beef, chicken or grilled veggies from last night. Feel free to add chorizo or bacon to double the taste.

Total Time Required

30-40 minutes

Nutritional Facts

Calories: 442
Cholesterol: 64mg
Carbohydrates: 31.88g
Protein: 9.74g
Fat: 32.02g

Ingredients

Tomato salsa (prepare by following the recipe above), 1 cup
Paleo-friendly tortilla chips (3 cups)
Homemade dairy-free sour cream (recipe above), ½ cup
Grass-fed goat grass fed cheese (grated), 1 cups
2 large-sized eggs

Ingredients for Garnish

Tomatoes (diced), ½ cup
Cilantro (chopped), ¼ cup
Avocado (diced), ½ cup

Grass-fed goat grass fed cheese (grated), ¼ cup
Red onion (mined), ¼ cup

Preparation Method

To prepare Chilaquiles, first prepare the tomato salsa, heat it and keep aside.

Set the oven to preheat at 350°F.

In a large skillet, combine tortilla chips (Paleo-friendly) and ¾ cup tomato salsa and toss to cover the chips. Add ½ cup grass fed cheese and ½ cup sour cream in the skillet and stir to combine.

Now transfer all the contents of the skillet in a greased baking dish and set to bake for 20 minutes until it's soft in the center and crispy on the edges.

Remove the baking dish, place the Chilaquiles on the plate and add the remaining grass fed cheese on the top. Set aside.

Before you serve, prepare eggs (the way you like) and place them over the Chilaquiles.

Last but not the least, garnish the dish with tomato, red onions, avocado, grass fed cheese and cilantro. Serve this delicious Mexican breakfast recipe hot on the table with extra salsa on the side.

Egg-Avocado Breakfast Burrito
Serves 4

Fresh, light and yet so filling. This incredible breakfast burrito recipe with authentic Mexican taste is the perfect way to kick-start your day. Make these lovely burritos at home for your breakfast and keep going throughout the day!

Total Time Required

35-40 minutes

Nutritional Facts

Calories: 460
Cholesterol: 235mg
Carbohydrates: 51g
Protein: 23g
Fat: 20g

Ingredients

Olive oil, 2 tsp
Red onion (diced), 1 cup
Red bell pepper, (diced and seeded), ½ cup
Chili flakes, ¼ tsp
Ground black pepper, to taste
Sea salt, to taste
Grass-fed goat grass fed cheese (shredded), ⅓ cup
4 Paleo-friendly tortillas (10" burrito size)
Salsa (your favorite), ¼ cup
4 eggs
4 egg whites only
Homemade dairy-free sour cream, ¼ cup
Tomato (seeded and diced), ½ cup
1 small-sized avocado (cubed)
Hot sauce (Paleo version)

Preparation Method

Set a non-stick skillet over med-high heat. Add olive oil to heat. add pepper and onions and cook for 6-8 minutes until onions are tender and peppers are charred. Add pepper flakes and cook for another few minutes. Season with pepper and salt and remove from heat. Shift all the contents into a dish.

In a bowl, whisk together eggs and egg whites. Stir in grass fed cheese and combine.

Grease the skillet with some oil and set it over med-high flame. After a few minutes, reduce heat to low and add the egg mixture. Scramble it by stirring occasionally for 2-3 minutes until cooked.

Spread a tablespoon of dairy-free sour cream on each tortilla and add salsa. Add the onion-pepper mixture next and finally add the scrambled eggs.

Garnish with avocado and diced tomatoes and season with hot sauce if you like. Wrap all 4 tortillas in a burrito-style and serve warm!

Ranch-Style Chicken Sandwich
Serves 4

Prepare the world's best Mexican chicken sandwich at home with this simple recipe. This is a basic recipe, you can always twist it up in your own personalized way by adding more ingredients such as chopped avocados, diced jalapenos or cilantro for added taste!

Total Time Required

32 minutes

Nutritional Facts

Calories: 614.2
Cholesterol: 118.4mg
Carbohydrates: 42.3g
Protein: 32.8g
Fat: 34.6g

Ingredients

Cream of chicken soup, 1 can
Homemade dairy-free sour cream, ½ cup
Grass-fed butter, 2 tbsp + more to grease grill pan
Onion (chopped), ½ cup
Chili powder, 1 tsp
Cooked chicken (diced), 2 cups
Green chilies (chopped), 1 can
Paleo-friendly tortillas, 8 pieces
Grass-fed goat grass fed cheese (in slices), 4 slices

Preparation Method

First of all, prepare tortillas.

Grease a grill pan with butter and roast tortilla on both sides for a minute. Once all are done, place them on a plate and set aside.

To prepare the sandwich filling, set the oven to preheat at 375°F.

In a small mixing bowl, add sour cream and cream of chicken sour and stir to mix.

Set a saucepan over low-med heat and add butter. Add onions and chili next and let it cook until onions are softened. Stir in chicken, 3 tbsp of soup/cream mixture and green chilies. When done, turn the stove off.

Place one tortilla on a plate, add a grass fed cheese slice and add 1 tbsp of soup/cream mix on top. Now add the chicken mixture on top and wrap it. Place another tortilla from the top and cover the open side of the tortilla to cover it up.

Prepare the remaining 3 sandwiches the same way and enjoy!

Mexican-Style Vegetable-Hotdog Burritos
Serves 4

Perfect recipe to prepare for that run in the morning! The blend of perfect Mexican flavors makes these burritos favorite among adults and children alike. Adjust the flavors, especially peppers according to your taste and you have the best Mexican-Style Vegetable Hotdog Burritos for the breakfast.

Total Time Required

50 minutes

Nutritional Facts

Calories: 212.4
Cholesterol: 116.7mg
Carbohydrates: 16g
Protein: 10.8g
Fat: 11.3g

Ingredients

2 eggs, beaten
Chunky salsa (any of your choice), ½ cup
High quality sausages (cooked and crumbled), ¼ lb
Grass-fed goat grass fed cheese (shredded), ½ cup
Paleo-friendly tortillas, 4 pieces
Green pepper (finely diced), ½ tbsp for each tortilla
¼ Jalapeno (sliced), to taste
1 small-sized red bell pepper (cut into strips)
1 small-sized yellow bell pepper (cut into strips)
1 small onion (chopped)
Tomatoes (peeled and chopped), ¼ cup

Preparation Method

Prepare scrambled eggs with two eggs in a large skillet. When done, stir in salsa and cooked, crumbled sausages.

Heat tortillas in a microwave for 20 seconds and set aside.

Place equal egg and hotdog mixture into 4 tortillas. Now add grass fed cheese, red pepper, jalapeno, onion, bell peppers and tomatoes on the top and wrap it up burrito style.

Set for another 20 seconds in the microwave and serve.

Note: Use only high quality hotdogs if you follow Paleo diet. Check for the ingredients in the label before picking one.

Hot Mexican Cocoa
Serves 3

Breakfast without a hot beverage is incomplete. And if you have Hot Mexican Cocoa on the menu, you will definitely want your hands on it. This recipe is particularly very popular among the little ones however, the inspiring taste will definitely impress the adults too. A must-try for a cold morning!

Total Time Required

10 minutes

Nutritional Facts

Calories: 184.7
Cholesterol: 26.5mg
Carbohydrates: 24.7g
Protein: 7.2g
Fat: 7.6g

Ingredients

Cocoa powder, 2 tbsp
Coconut milk, 2 ½ cups
Pure vanilla extract, ½ tsp
Ground cinnamon, ¼ tsp
Raw honey, 2 tbsp
Pure maple syrup, 1 tbsp
Dark chocolate (crushed), for garnish

Preparation Method

Set a non-stick saucepan over low-med heat. Add cocoa, maple syrup, hone and cinnamon. Stir to combine.

Next, add coconut milk and stir constantly until all the ingredients are combined well. Let the mixture heat at medium flame. Do not boil.

Turn off the stove and stir in vanilla extract. Let it cool a bit. Beat with an electric mixer until the mixture is frothy. Pour into cups. Garnish with crushed dark chocolate and serve immediately.

Mexican Lunch: Peppery, Pleasant Meals

Are you ready to prepare the best Mexican dishes for lunch? Lunch time is the trickiest time of all to come up with a recipe that kids and adults would enjoy. With the range of Mexican recipes shared here, you can now enjoy a new Mexican recipe every day.

Here's your chance to become an expert Mexican chef, without stepping out of your house and without cheating on your Paleo lifestyle. Check out these recipes below:

Chicken Chili Quesadilla
Serves 8

Prepare this simple recipe with flour-free tortillas. Just a handful of ingredients are enough to prepare these delicious quesadillas in the perfect Mexican way. Serve with your favorite salsa (you can use to make one using the recipes shared above). Enjoy warm!

Total Time Required

20 minutes

Nutritional Facts

Calories: 290.8
Cholesterol: 42.2mg
Carbohydrates: 26g
Protein: 11.3g
Fat: 16g

Ingredients

Tortillas (Paleo-friendly), 8 pieces (burrito style)
Grass-fed goat grass fed cheese (finely shredded), 2 cups
4 green chilies (chopped)
Cooked chicken (finely chopped), 2 cups
Grass-fed butter (melted), 2 tbsp
Salsa (your favorite), 1 cup

Preparation Method

Place a tortilla on a plate. Cover half of it with grass fed cheese, green chilies and chicken. Fold the other half to cover the filling. Press to adjust properly. Set the filling in each of the 8 tortillas.

Set a nonstick skillet over low-med heat.

Meanwhile, brush all the tortillas with butter and set aside. Now place them in the skillet in a batch of 2-3 and cook for 3-4 minutes, turning just once. When the tortillas turn golden brown, remove from the skillet and place it in a pan.

Slice it into wedges. Prepare the remaining tortillas the same way.

Serve with your favorite salsa and enjoy!

Beefy Enchiladas
Serves 4-6

A plate full of flavors. You cannot say no to Mexican Beefy Enchiladas. The recipe not only tastes delicious but looks so appetizing that you will not be able to keep your hands off it. 45 minutes is all that it takes to prepare this cheesy, mouthwatering Mexican Paleo dish.

Total Time Required

45 minutes

Nutritional Facts

Calories: 740.5
Cholesterol: 131.3mg
Carbohydrates: 51.8g
Protein: 44.3g
Fat: 40.2g

Ingredients

Ground beef, 1 lb
Onion (chopped), ¼ cup
Garlic powder, 1 tsp
Tomato sauce, 1 can
Paprika, 1 tsp
Chili powder, 2 tsp
Oregano, 1 tsp
Grass-fed goat grass fed cheese (shredded), 3 cups
Black pepper, ½ tsp
12 Paleo-friendly tortillas
Enchilada sauce (green), 1 can
Black olives (sliced), 1 cup
Olive oil

Preparation Method

Heat oil in a skillet over low-med flame. Add onion followed by garlic. Add ground beef next and fry until brown. Cook for a few minutes then add tomato sauce, paprika, oregano, chili powder, cumin and black pepper. Stir and cook until the beef is done. Remove and set aside.

In another skillet, add oil and heat. Place tortillas in the skillet, cooking for 10 seconds per side. Remove and drain the oil on a paper towel. Repeat with the remaining tortillas.

Prepare a baking pan. Add enchilada sauce and cover the bottom of the pan. Add the meat mixture to each tortilla along with 1 tbsp grass fed cheese, chopped onions and some olives. Roll it up and place it in the baking sheet with seam side down. Repeat with the remaining tortillas and fill the pan.

Pour some enchilada sauce over tortillas and cover it up with the remaining grass fed cheese and olives.

Set to bake for 20 minutes at 350°F. When done remove and allow to cool slightly. Cut into pieces before you serve. Add homemade dairy-free sour cream from the top and enjoy!

Salsa in Chicken Burritos
Serves 2

Burritos, one of the most popular part of the Mexican cuisine can be made with different types of fillings. This particular burrito is unique with its unique taste of grilled chicken along with a mix of two different salsas. Enjoy the hot, pepper flavors wrapped in a tortilla for you. Serve warm.

Total Time Required

20 minutes

Nutritional Facts

Calories: 766.6
Cholesterol: 101.8mg
Carbohydrates: 79.2g
Protein: 48.2g
Fat: 27.8g

Ingredients

Chicken breast (grilled, flattened and cut in strips), 1 cup
Salsa (your favorite), ⅔ cups
Squash pasta sauce, 1/3 cup
Hot salsa, ¼ cup
Tortillas (Paleo-friendly), 2 large
Grass-fed goat grass fed cheese (grated), ½ cup
Homemade dairy-free sour cream, 2 tbsp

Preparation Method

In a mixing bowl, add chicken strips along with squash pasta sauce and toss to combine flavors. Let it sit for 10 minutes.

Meanwhile, in another bowl, combine salsa and hot salsa together.

Now spread 2 large tortillas in two plates. Divide the chicken into half and place it on the tortillas. Similarly, divide the salsa mix into half too and spread over the chicken equally. Sprinkle grass fed cheese equally on both the tortillas.

Roll them up and set them on a baking sheet with the seam side down. Set to bake for 5-6 minutes at 375°F. When done, remove from the oven and add a dollop of homemade dairy-free sour cream on the tortillas. Serve warm and enjoy!

Tasty Taco Casserole
Serves 6-8

With tortilla chips on the bottom and different layers of beef, veggies, seasoning and lots of grass fed cheese, this dish will be a super-hit amongst children and adults alike as you serve Taco Casserole for lunch. Adjust the flavors and add more salsa, grass fed cheese and olives as you like.

Total Time Required

30 minutes

Nutritional Facts

Calories: 349.9
Cholesterol: 72.8mg
Carbohydrates: 16.2g
Protein: 24.1g
Fat: 21.3g

Ingredients

Ground beef, 1 lb
Taco seasoning (Paleo-version), 1 package
Grass-fed goat grass fed cheese, 2 cups (divided)
Green onions (chopped), ¼ cup
Salsa (any of your choice), 1 cup
Black olives (sliced), 1 cup
1 large tomato (chopped)
Tortilla chips (Paleo friendly), 2 cups

Preparation Method

Add ground beef in a large, non-stick skillet and cook until brown. Drain.

Add taco seasoning in the beef and cook for another few minutes, adding water as required by the package directions.

Cover the bottom of 8x8 baking dish with tortilla chips. Melt grass fed cheese and mix with salsa. Pour this mixture over the chips. Add beef on top and cover with the remaining 1 cup grass fed cheese on the top. Sprinkle olives and green onions over grass fed cheese.

Set to bake for 8-10 minutes at 375°F, until the grass fed cheese is completely melted.

Remove from the oven and add thinly chopped tomatoes on the top. Let it cool for a few minutes and then serve warm.

Juicy Wet Burritos
Serves 4

Mexican cuisine is all about different flavors and types of burritos. Even if you are following a Paleo diet, you can enjoy a variety of burritos that you can prepare at home. This recipe includes several ingredients to give this dish its unique flavors. Feel free to use chicken instead of beef if you like. The gravy from the top will make these burritos very juicy and tender.

Total Time Required

35 minutes

Nutritional Facts

Calories: 1028.4
Cholesterol: 136.8mg
Carbohydrates: 98.3g
Protein: 60.2g
Fat: 43.9g

Ingredients

Ground beef, 1 lb
Garlic (pressed), 2 cloves
Paprika, 1 tsp
Onion (finely chopped), ½ cup
Mexican oregano, 1 tsp
Cumin, ¾ tsp
Chili powder, 1 ½ tsp
Black pepper, ½ tsp
Tomatoes (diced), 1 cup
Flour-less tortillas, 4 large-sized
Enchilada sauce, 1 can of 10 oz
Homemade beef gravy, 1 jar of 18 oz
Grass-fed goat grass fed cheese (shredded), 2 cups

Ingredients for Serving

Chopped onion, ¼ cup
Homemade dairy-free sour cream, ½ cup
Jalapeno (thinly sliced), a few
Salsa of your choice, 1 cup

1 medium-sized tomato (chopped)
Lettuce (chopped), ½ cup

Preparation Method

Brown beef with garlic and onion and cook for a few minutes. Drain to remove the fat from browning.

In the same skillet, add paprika, chili powder, oregano, half of the tomatoes and pepper and combine. Let the ingredients simmer for 4-5 minutes.

While the meat is simmering, prepare the gravy by combining beef gravy, enchilada sauce, and the remaining tomatoes. Cook until the mixture starts boiling.

Follow the package directions to soften tortillas.

Set the oven to preheat at 375°F.

To assemble burritos, place a tortilla and spread ¼ of the meat mixture over it. Add ¼ cup grass fed cheese on the top and roll from both the ends to close it. Place it seam side down on a prepared baking dish.

Repeat the process with remaining tortillas and assemble them on the baking dish and set to bake for 15-20 minutes until the burritos are thoroughly heated and the grass fed cheese is melted.

When done, remove from the oven, transfer the burritos on a serving plate and spoon the gravy/sauce you prepared over the top.

Garnish with chopped tomatoes, lettuce, jalapenos, onions and lots of sour cream and salsa on the side as you desire.

Mexican Taco Bell Pizza

Serves 4

Don't miss this amazing Mexican pizza recipe and enjoy a delicious Mexican cuisine on your lunch table. With layers of Paleo-friendly tortillas, meat, vegetables and salsa seasoning, this recipe will serve your taste buds with exotic flavors.

Total Time Required

30 minutes

Nutritional Facts

Calories: 905.5
Cholesterol: 93.5mg
Carbohydrates: 53.5g
Protein: 36.7g
Fat: 88g

Ingredients

Ground beef, ½ lb
Sea salt, ½ tsp
Paprika, ¼ paprika
Onion (minced), ¼ tsp
Water, 2 tbsp
Chili powder, 1 ½ tsp
8 large tortillas (flour-free)
Tomato (diced), ⅓ cup
Picante sauce (mild), ⅔ cup
Olive oil, 1 cup
Grass-fed goat grass fed cheese (shredded), 2 cup
Green onion (chopped), ¼ cup
Bell peppers (chopped), 1 cup
Black olives (sliced), ¼ cup
Salsa (your favorite), 1 cup

Preparation Method

Cook beef over low-medium heat. When done, drain and place the meat back to pan. Add salt, paprika, onions, water and chili powder. Combine and let the mixture simmer over low heat for 5-10 minutes. Constantly stir while the mixture simmers.

Meanwhile, set a frying pan over med-high heat and add oil. When oil is hot, toss tortillas and cook on both the sides for a few seconds. Remove and drain on paper towels and repeat with the remaining tortillas.

Fry tortillas until golden brown, do not let any bubbles pop.

Set the oven to preheat at 400°F.

Place one tortilla on a plate and spread the meat evenly. Place another tortilla and cover with a layer of your favorite salsa. Divide and add tomatoes, bell peppers, olives, onions and cover with grass fed cheese. Set to bake for 10-12 minutes until the grass fed cheese melts and ingredients tenderize.

Repeat with the remaining tortillas and enjoy this amazing, Mexican taco bell pizza

Serves 4

All these delicious, authentic Mexican flavors can be blended into one recipe to prepare a peppery fajita. Savor this amazing recipe with grilled chicken, bell peppers, and vegetable sauce with vinegar, liquid smoke and garlic. Serve hot and enjoy.

Total Time Required

4 hours

Nutritional Facts

Calories: 132.3
Cholesterol: 0mg
Carbohydrates: 9.8g
Protein: 1.7g
Fat: 10.3g

Ingredients

Chicken breast (skinless, boneless), 1 lb
1 large-sized Spanish onion (thinly sliced)
½ green bell pepper (thinly sliced)
½ red bell pepper (thinly sliced)
½ yellow bell pepper (thinly sliced)

Ingredients for Marinade

Lime juice, ¼ cup
Water, ⅓ cup
Olive oil, 2 tbsp
Sea salt, 1 tsp
Garlic (crushed), 4 cloves
Liquid smoke, ½ tsp
Black pepper, ¼ tsp
Cayenne pepper 1/2 tsp

Ingredients for Vegetable Sauce

Water, 1 tbsp
Lime juice, ½ tsp
Olive oil, 1 tbsp
Vinegar, 1 tsp

Sea salt, a dash
Black pepper, a dash

Preparation Method

In a Tupperware container, combine water, juice, garlic, oil, salt, cayenne pepper, liquid smoke, black pepper with chicken. Mix to combine flavors. Cover and set to refrigerate for at least 2 hours or overnight.

When done, grill chicken over low-med flame for 5-8 minutes, cooking on each side. When cooked, remove and place it on a cutting board. Let it cool slightly and then cut thin strips. Keep warm and set aside.

In a bowl, combine vinegar, water, salt, olive oil, pepper and lime juice. Set aside.

In a pan, cook peppers and onion in hot oil for a few minutes until tender and brown. Remove and place it on a serving dish. Pour the vegetable mixture over the peppers, combine meat, peppers, onions and serve hot.

Mexican Chicken Squash pasta
Serves 6

Serve hot the best-tasting Mexican squash pasta, which you can prepare within 35 minutes, on your lunch table. With the most common ingredients your pantry is stocked with, you can prepare easy-to-make, juicy, and very affordable squash pasta in no time. Serve hot.

Total Time Required

35 minutes

Nutritional Facts

Calories: 321.1
Cholesterol: 24.2mg
Carbohydrates: 49g
Protein: 19.6g
Fat: 5.3g

Ingredients

Chicken broth (low-sodium), 4 cups
Garlic (minced), 1 clove
Chili powder, ½ tsp
Cumin,1 tsp
6 tomatoes
3 scallions
1 large-sized bell pepper (green)
Vermicelli, ¾ lb
Chicken breast (skinless, boneless), ½ lb
Olive oil, 1 tbsp
Green chilies (mild), 2 tbsp
Sea salt,1/4 tsp
Fresh cilantro (chopped), ¼ cup

Preparation Method

Place a medium-sized saucepan over med-high heat. Add chicken broth, chili powder, cumin and garlic. Stir and bring the mixture to boil.

Meanwhile, chop bell pepper, scallion and tomatoes and set aside. Break vermicelli into small pieces (2-inch).

Add chicken in the broth mixture and reduce the heat. Cover the saucepan and let it simmer for 8-10 minutes until chicken is thoroughly cooked. When done, remove chicken from the broth and let it cool. Set aside.

In a large skillet, heat oil over med-high flame. Add vermicelli and cook. Stir constantly and cook for 2-3 minutes until it is browned.

Add the broth mixture, scallions, tomatoes, green chilies, bell pepper and sea salt and bring to boil again over med heat. After a few minutes, reduce heat and cover the skillet. Let it simmer, stir and cook for another 5-7 minutes until the squash pasta is done.

Meanwhile, thinly chop cilantro and shred chicken. Stir in cilantro and shredded chicken into the skillet and combine with the squash pasta mixture. When done, turn off the stove and serve hot.

Mexican Dinner – Delicious Tex-Mex Menu

A range of Mexican recipes can be prepared especially for dinner. This authentic tex-mex menu can be prepared for your family or bunch of friends coming over for a Mexican-themed party.

Serve hot and blend the peppery ingredients together to enjoy the authentic flavors of Mexico. Check out the recipes below:

Mexican Stew
Serves 5

Stews can be made Mexican style too! Just grab a few ingredients listed below and prepare delicious chicken stew. 30 minutes is all that it takes to prepare a delicious, peppery Mexican recipe to savor with everyone else on the dining table.

Total Time Required

30 minutes

Nutritional Facts

Calories: 359.3
Cholesterol: 63mg
Carbohydrates: 39.8g
Protein: 30.8g
Fat: 9.7g

Ingredients

Onion (diced), 1 cup
Garlic (finely chopped), 2 cloves
Olive oil, 1 tbsp
Chicken (cooked and diced), 3 cups
Tomatoes (diced), 1 ½ cups
Taco seasoning mix (Paleo-friendly), 1 package
Green chilies (diced), 1 can of 4 oz
Chicken broth, 1 cup

Preparation Method

Set a saucepan over low-med heat and add oil. Stir in onion and garlic and cook. When onions are tender, add chicken, tomatoes, taco seasoning and chilies.

Add broth to the saucepan and stir with the remaining ingredients. Bring the mixture to boil, reduce heat and simmer for 10-15 minutes. Make sure you stir occasionally to combine the ingredients well.

Your stew is now ready to be served.

Mexican Steak Fajita
Serves 8

Tender beef steak, saucy mixtures and ample of choices for toppings, prepare Mexican steak fajita just the right way with this recipe. Add your personalized touch to this recipe by using any combination of the toppings from the list or all of them for enhanced flavors.

Total Time Required

20 minutes

Nutritional Facts

Calories: 137.1
Cholesterol: 0mg
Carbohydrates: 18.3g
Protein: 2.9g
Fat: 5.8g

Ingredients

Top sirloin steak, ¾ lb
Olive oil, 2 tbsp
Lime juice, 1 tbsp
Garlic (minced), 1 clove
Chili powder ½ tsp
Cumin, ½ tsp
Hot pepper flakes, ½ tsp
Sea salt, ½ tsp
8 flourless tortillas (8 inch)
Onion (chopped), ½ cup
2 small-sized sweet peppers (yellow, red or green)

Ingredients for Topping

Salsa of your choice, 1 cup
Homemade dairy-free sour cream, 1 cup
Grass-fed goat grass fed cheese, 1 cup
1 large-sized tomato (chopped)

Preparation Method

Cut steaks into strips (thin).

In a mixing bowl, add 1 tbsp oil, garlic, lime juice, cumin, chili powder, salt, black pepper and hot pepper flakes. Add steak strips into the mixture and combine to coat. Let it sit in the bowl for a few minutes.

Meanwhile, roll tortillas in foil and set to heat for 5-8 minutes at 350°F until heated and tender.

Thinly slice onions into strips and cut peppers in a similar way.

Heat olive oil (remaining 1 tbsp) in a skillet over med-high heat. Add sliced peppers and onions and stir constantly for 2-4 minutes until tender. When done, remove and place in a bowl.

Add the mixture-coated beef strips into the skillet and cook for a few minutes, stirring constantly. When the color changes to brown, stir in pepper and onions to the skillet again. Stir and cook for another 1 minute. When the beef is done, turn off the stove.

To serve, place one tortilla on a plate and spoon some beef right in the centre, add all the divided toppings one by one and cover the tortilla. Repeat with the remaining tortillas and serve warm.

Savory Manicotti
Serves 8

Prepare Savory Manicotti without the manincotti shell. This special Paleo Mexican recipe can be made without the forbidden ingredient replaced by flourless, Paleo-friendly tortillas. The blend of sauce and grass fed cheese with onions and olives will make this recipe very unique and flavorful. Enjoy!

Total Time Required
1 hour 30 minutes

Nutritional Facts

Calories: 449.5
Cholesterol: 80.5mg
Carbohydrates: 36.3g
Protein: 23.9g
Fat: 23.5g

Ingredients

Ground beef, 1 lb
Chili powder, 1 can of 16 oz
Oregano, 3 tsp
Water, 2 ½ cups
8 flourless tortillas
Picante sauce, 16 oz
Grass-fed goat grass fed cheese (shredded), 1 cup
Homemade dairy-free sour cream, 1 cup
Green onions (sliced), ¼ cup
Black olives (sliced), ¼ cup

Preparation Method

Mix beef, oregano and chili powder in a mixing bowl. Spoon this mixture into heated tortillas. Prepare all the tortillas likewise.

Prepare a baking pan (13x9 inches) and grease it with olive oil.

Mix sauce and water in a bowl and pour over the tortilla manicotti. If you like, add chopped cilantro on the top.

Cover the baking pan with plastic wraps and set to refrigerate for at least 8 hours to overnight.

Before you set to bake it, remove at least 30 minutes before.

Set to bake the tortilla manicotti (covered) for 60 minutes at 350°F.

When done remove from the oven and uncover. Sprinkle with olives, onions and grass fed cheese. Set to bake for another 8 to 10 minutes (uncovered).

Serve hot with sour cream on the side.

Mexican Shrimp Cocktail
Serves 4-6

Dipped in an interesting homemade Mexican sauce, enjoy crunchy shrimp in the real Mexican flavors. Serve them in the cocktail glass or present them on a plate with sauce and garnishes on top, either way the flavors will give you a very unique dining experience.

Total Time Required

2 hour 15 minutes

Nutritional Facts

Calories: 386.1
Cholesterol: 442mg
Carbohydrates: 23.8g
Protein: 49.8g
Fat: 10.2g

Ingredients

Shrimp (deveined, peeled and cooked), 2 lbs
Garlic (crushed), 1 tbsp
Red onion (finely chopped), ½ cup
Fresh cilantro, ¼ cup
Clamato juice, 1 ½ cups
Ketchup, ¼ cup
Lime juice (fresh), ¼ cup
1 Serrano pepper (minced)
Prepared horseradish, ¼ cup
Sea salt, to taste
1 medium-sized Avocado (pitted, peeled and chopped)

Preparation Method

Place cooked shrimp in a large bowl.

Add cilantro, red onion and garlic. Mix to combine.

Stir in horseradish, Serrano, limejuice, ketchup, and Clamato. Sprinkle salt to season. Toss to combine all the flavors. Cover with plastic wrap and set to refrigerate for 2-3 hours.

To serve, first add fresh avocado and then enjoy the unique flavors of Mexican-style shrimp cocktail with friends and family.

Jalapeno Mexican Burger
Serves 6

Prepare caramelized jalapeno and onion relish and red-pepper mayonnaise paste before you set to prepare the burgers to give this recipe the authentic Mexican flavors it deserves. With patties made of beef and chorizos, these hamburger rolls will take you to a different world of Mexican flavors you will fall in love with.

Total Time Required
1 hour 10 minutes

Nutritional Facts

Calories: 395.2
Cholesterol: 58.1mg
Carbohydrates: 19.4g
Protein: 32g
Fat: 7.7g

Ingredients

Ground sirloin, ¾ lb
Beef steak, ¾ lb
Raw chorizo (crumbled, casings removed), ½ lb
Adobo seasoning, 1 tbsp
Bread crumbs (Paleo version), ½ cup
1 large-sized onion (grated)
Olive oil, 2 tbsp
2 large-sized yellow onions (thinly sliced)
Jalapeno chilies (sliced), ½ cup
Sea salt, to taste
Ground black pepper, to taste
Dark brown sugar, ½ cup
Homemade dairy-free mayonnaise, ¾ cup
2 medium-sized red bell peppers (roasted)
Grass-fed goat grass fed cheese, 6 slices
Paleo-friendly hamburger rolls, 6 pieces

Preparation Method

In a large-sized mixing bowl, add chorizo, ground beef, bread crumbs, onion and adobo seasoning and mix well using your hand. Now use the mixture to form six beef patties for the burgers.

Prepare a baking dish and layer with wax paper. Place the patties, cover with plastic wrap and set to refrigerate for 30 minutes.

Meanwhile, prepare caramelized jalapeno and onion relish. Set a large skillet over low-med heat and add olive oil. Add onion in hot oil and seasons with pepper and salt, stirring. Next, add jalapenos followed by brown sugar. Stir constantly to sauté the ingredients together. Cook for 15 minutes and chilies and onions are tender and thoroughly caramelized. When done, remove and set aside.

Next, prepare red-pepper mayonnaise. Place the roasted red bell peppers in a food processor or blender. Sprinkle some salt and pepper and mayonnaise. Pulse all the ingredients together to prepare a well-mixed, smooth puree. Set into the refrigerator to chill until you are ready to use it.

The final step is to prepare the Jalapeno Mexican Burgers. Preheat the grill pan or an outdoor grill over med-high heat. Place the patties on the grill pan/outdoor grill and cook until the desired doneness. Cook for at least 5 minutes on each side.

Just before you are ready to remove the patties, place 1 slice grass fed cheese on each patty and let it melt. Remove and set aside. Cook all the patties likewise.

To serve, first prepare the hamburger rolls. Spread red-pepper mayonnaise puree on both the sides evenly. Place the patty on the bottom half and cover it with lots of jalapeno and onion caramelized relish. Repeat for the remaining burgers and serve hot.

Short Mexican BBQ Ribs
Serves 8

Salt, pepper, red wine vinegar and a cup filled with tomatillo salsa – everything you need to give the beef short ribs its best flavors. With as few as four ingredients, you can enjoy a meal at dinner that your family will relish. Grill the ribs on gas or over charcoal, you will definitely love with the authentic taste of this simple recipe.

Total Time Required
1 hour 20 minutes

Nutritional Facts

Calories: 510.3
Cholesterol: 65.1mg
Carbohydrates: 24.2g
Protein: 33g
Fat: 8.7g

Ingredients

Beef short ribs (cut into thick slices), 4lb
Sea salt, to taste
Ground black pepper, to taste
Red wine vinegar
Tomatillo Salsa, 2 cups

Preparation Method

Clear fat from the beef ribs. Sprinkle salt and pepper and rub over the meat surface generously to coat. Place the beef ribs in a greased baking dish and adjust them in a single layer. Add vinegar on top and turn to cover them with vinegar on both the side.

Let it sit for at least 1 hour (you can choose to keep for up to 4 hours if you have time). Turn occasionally to allow the ribs absorb flavors nicely.

Depending on how you would like to cook the ribs, build proper charcoal fire or set the gas grill to preheat at med-high heat.

Set the ribs to cook, turning them only once on the grill when it is well browned on all sides. It is recommended to cook at least 6 minutes per side. When done on both sides, remove and serve it on a plate. Allow to cool for a few minutes before serving them for dinner along with tomatillo salsa (recipe above).

Enjoy!

Mexican Creamy Lasagna
Serves 8

Who said you cannot enjoy a creamy, cheesy lasagna when following Paleo diet? The Mexican menu allows you to enjoy lasagna without involving any restricted ingredient. Add flour-less tortillas instead of lasagna sheets and enjoy the authentic flavor by using grass-fed goat grass fed cheese instead of regular one. Must-try this delicious recipe!

Total Time Required
45 minutes

Nutritional Facts

Calories: 219.2
Cholesterol: 42.6mg
Carbohydrates: 21.2g
Protein: 21.3g
Fat: 6.3g

Ingredients

Ground turkey, 1 lb
Taco seasoning (Paleo friendly), 1 package of 2 oz.
Onion (chopped), ½ cup
Tomato sauce (low-sodium), 1 ½ cups
Fresh tomato salsa (1 cup)
Grass-fed goat grass fed cheese, 2 cups
4 eggs
Flour-free tortillas, 8 pieces
Olives (slices), ½ cup

Preparation Method

Set the oven to preheat at 350°F.

Brown ground turkey and drain if required.

Add tomato salsa, sauce, onion and taco seasoning. Combine and let the mixture simmer for 5-6 minutes.

In a small bowl, mix egg and 1 cup grass fed cheese together.

Prepare a baking sheet and grease it with olive oil or cooking spray.

Place ½ meat mixture, 4 pieces of tortillas, ½ cup grass fed cheese mixture, ½ cup grass fed cheese. Repeat the same order to form another layer. Add slices olives in the end.

Set to bake for 25 minutes or more, until the grass fed cheese melts. When done, remove and allow to cool. Enjoy the cheesy Mexican lasagna.

Seafood Stew with Lime and Tomatoes
Serves 4-6

Enhance the combination of seafood specialties by adding lime and tomatoes. Prepare the recipes on time and served with flour-less tortillas, lime wedges, avocado and coriander for amazing flavors. Enjoy special Mexican seafood stew like never before.

Total Time Required

45 minutes

Nutritional Facts

Calories: 347
Cholesterol: 8.9mg
Carbohydrates: 28g
Protein: 44g
Fat: 6g

Ingredients

2 Guajillo chili (dried)
Olive oil, 1 tbsp
1 large-sized onion (finely chopped)
Chipotle paste, 1 tsp
Ground cumin, 1 tsp
Chicken stock, 3 cups
Tomatoes (chopped), 1 cup
Prawns (peeled), 1 cup
Fish fillets (cut into small 2 ½ cm pieces), 1 ½ cups
Clams, 1 cup
Potatoes (sliced into halves and boiled), 2 cups
lime juice, 2 tbsp
Salt, to taste
Black pepper, to taste

To Serve

1 avocado (thinly chopped)
Lime wedges
Coriander leaves, a handful
Red onion (finely diced), 2 tbsp
Flourless tortillas, baked and sliced

Preparation Method

In a hot frying pan, toast chilies dry until they puff a little. Remove from pan, stem chilies and deseed them. Next, soak them in boiling water for 10 to 15 minutes.

Meanwhile, set a large saucepan over low-med flame and heat olive oil. Add onion and garlic and season with salt and pepper. Cook until tender. Add reconstituted chilies, chipotle paste, tomatoes, cumin and stock. Combine and sauté for 4-5 minutes.

Transfer all the ingredients into a heat-resistant blender and pulse to puree. When done, pour the mixture back into the pan and let it boil. Reduce the heat to low and let it simmer for 10-12 minutes.

Before serving, add clams, fish fillets, prawns and potatoes. Cover the pan and cook for 5 minutes. Add lime juice and stir. Serve with tortilla chips, red onion, coriander, avocado and lime wedges. Enjoy!

Vegetarian Chili
Serves 12

This recipe brings all the authentic vegetables and peppery flavors together! The perfect vegetarian chili you enjoy at restaurants can now be prepared at home, with simple ingredients you already have in your pantry. Feel free to adjust the chili if you want your children to enjoy equally.

Total Time Required
45 minutes

Nutritional Facts

Calories: 184.6
Cholesterol: 0mg
Carbohydrates: 31.1g
Protein: 8.2g
Fat: 4.5g

Ingredients

2 medium-sized zucchini (chopped)
Green pepper (chopped), 1 cup
1 medium-sized onion (chopped)
Sweet red pepper (chopped), 1 cup
Garlic (minced), 3 cloves
Olive oil, 3 tbsp
Italian stewed tomatoes (cut into small pieces), 2 cans
Tomato sauce, 1 can
1 jalapeno pepper (chopped and seeded)
Fresh cilantro (minced), ¼ cup
Fresh parsley (minced), ¼ cup
Chili powder, 3 tbsp
Raw honey, 4 tbsp
Sea salt, 1 tsp
Ground cumin, 1 tsp

Preparation Method

Place a large pot over low-med heat. Add oil and heat. Stir in zucchini, peppers, onion and garlic and cook until tender. Keep stirring.

Next, add all the remaining ingredients including stewed tomatoes, tomato sauce, jalapeno, parsley, cilantro, honey, chili powder, cumin and salt. Stir to combine flavors and cook until it boils.

Reduce the flame, cover the pot and let the mixture simmer for another 30 minutes. Stir occasionally until done.

Remove from heat and serve hot.

Mexican Desserts – Sweet Something

Some of the best tasting desserts and candies are Mexican. Even if you are following a Paleo diet that restricts the consumption of sugar and flour, you still have many options left that you can try at home and serve your sweet taste buds.

No more 'sweets' deprived. With Paleo Mexican dessert recipes we have shared with you here, you can prepare the best of recipes without cheating on your diet. Check out yourself and enjoy the best Mexican desserts at home.

Mexican Crullers
Serves 10-12 (24 churros)

The famous Mexican crullers recipe has been adjusted to fulfill your Paleo needs. Enjoy the authentic taste of Mexican crullers with this amazing recipe. Feel free to shape your crullers are you like. Make long strips or make a cruller flower for your little ones. This recipe welcomes some amazing creativity. Enjoy!

Total Time Required
30 minutes

Nutritional Facts

Calories: 26.9
Cholesterol: 15.5mg
Carbohydrates: 4.5g
Protein: 1g
Fat: 0.4g

Ingredients

Water, 1 cup
Raw honey, 2 tbsp
Pure maple syrup, 1 tbsp
Sea salt, 1 tsp
Blanched almond flour, 1 cup
2 eggs
½ rind of lemon
Olive oil, for frying
Coconut sugar (powdered), ¼ cup

Preparation Method

Combine water, salt, maple syrup and honey in a bowl. Transfer to a small pot and bring the mixture to boil over low-med heat. When done, remove from heat.

Stir in almond flour at once and beat to prepare a smooth mixture. You can do it using an electric hand mixture. Add one egg and beat along. Add another after a while and keep beating the mixture until smooth.

Time to prepare the Mexican Crullers! Add this mixture into a pastry bag with a large, star-shaped opening. Now make strips (not more than 3 inches) with the mixture on a large, flat baking dish with either floured surface or covered with wax paper.

In a large, nonstick frying pan, add olive oil or fat for frying. Add lemon peel. When the oil or fat is hot, add a few crullers at a time and cook until the color changes to golden for 3-4 minutes. Turn to cook on all sides.

Remove and place it on paper towels to drain. Roll in coconut sugar immediately.

Repeat with the remaining and serve the delicious, Mexican crullers.

Chili Chocolate Cake
Serves 12

The unique sweet and peppery flavors definitely make this dessert recipe worth trying. You can adjust the peppery flavor by reducing the amount of chilies and red pepper flakes used if you only want a hint of chili. This authentic Mexican dessert will leave your taste buds confused with the best of flavors lingering for longer than you expect.

Total Time Required

1 hour 30 minutes

Nutritional Facts

Calories: 105
Cholesterol: 25mg
Carbohydrates: 19g
Protein: 4.1g
Fat: 5.4g

Ingredients for the Sponge

Blanched almond flour, 1 cup
Brown sugar, ½ cup
Pure maple syrup, ¼ cup
Grass-fed unsalted butter, 1 cup
3 eggs (beaten)
Cocoa powder, 2 tbsp
Baking powder, 1 tsp
1 red chili pepper (minced), choose mild, sweet chilies instead of fiery ones
Chili flakes (dried), ½ tsp

Ingredients for Frosting and Filling

Dark chocolate, 1 ½ cups
Homemade dairy-free sour cream, ½ cup
Grass fed unsalted butter, 2 tbsp
1 red chili pepper (minced)
Hot chili powder, ½ tsp
Chili flakes (dried), ½ tsp

Preparation Method

Add cocoa powder, almond flour and baking powder in a mixing bowl and combine. Add brown sugar, maple syrup, eggs, butter, dried and fresh chili in the dry mixture and beat thoroughly to make a soft, smooth wet mixture.

If your mixture is too thick or stiff, add a few drops of water. Add the mixture into a greased large cake tin. Smooth the top using a spatula or spoon. Set to bake for 30 minutes at 325°F. Check for doneness by inserting a knife. When done, remove from the oven and allow to cool (for up to an hour).

Meanwhile, prepare your filling and frosting. First of all, melt the chocolate (either using a double boiler or place it in a microwave for a minute or two). Stir in cream, butter and chilies in the chocolate. Cover the bowl with cling film and set to cool. When cooled, place in the refrigerator to adjust the consistency. Make sure it doesn't get too hard to spread.

Slice your cake into two equal halves right from the center. Lift the top part carefully and spread the chocolate filling and spread with a knife or spoon. Place the top back on its place and cover the top with the remaining frosting. Decorate with fresh and dried red chilies and enjoy.

Mexican Grass fed cheesecake
Serves 10-12

Mexican grass fed cheesecake with blueberry flavor detailing is finger-licking good. The soft custardy flan could take several steps to prepare, but every minute is worth spending if you are getting Mexican grass fed cheesecake to enjoy at the end. Your kids will love you for this!

Total Time Required
1 hour (inactive preparation time is 2 hours)

Nutritional Facts

Calories: 310.8
Cholesterol: 120.9mg
Carbohydrates: 37.5g
Protein: 9g
Fat: 14.2g

Ingredients

Pure maple syrup, 4 tbsp
Water, ¼ cup
Cream grass fed cheese (dairy-free), 12 oz
3 large-sized eggs
Almond milk, 2 cups
Coconut milk (evaporated), 1 cup
Raw honey, ½ cup
Vanilla extract, 1 tsp
Blueberries (fresh), 1 cup

Preparation Method

Fill a large bowl with ice water and place it near your stove.

Set a medium saucepan over med-high heat. Add ¼ cup water along with maple syrup. Stir to dissolve it completely. Swirl the saucepan a few times. Cook the mixture for 10 minutes.

Place the saucepan in the ice water to discontinue the cooking completely. Pour this maple-caramel mixture in 10-12 prepared ramekins. Set aside.

Set your oven to preheat at 325°F.

In a bowl, add eggs and cream grass fed cheese and beat using an electric hand mixer. Increase the speed to combine the ingredients well. Add honey, coconut milk, almond milk and vanilla extract and beat again until all ingredients are combined together.

Now add this custard over the caramel you have already added into the ramekins. When all the ramekins are done, prepare the roasting pan by placing a kitchen towel on it and place ramekins in two rows. Now add hot water into the baking dish until it reaches halfway up the ramekins.

Cover the roasting pan or baking dish with tight aluminum foil and set to bake for around 30 minutes. Check if the flans are still wobbly as you touch the edges.

When done, place the baking dish on a slap. Remove the foil and allow to cool. Remove ramekins from water (be very careful while handling it). Allow it to cool for another few minutes. You can refrigerate the flans for up to 4 days before serving, if you like.

Before serving, run a knife around the ramekin edge to loosen the custard flan. Place it on a plate upside down to invert onto a serving plate. Serve with fresh blueberries for enhanced flavors.

Serves 12

Chocolate on the bottom – chocolate on the top! With the base and topping both made from the authentic flavors of dark chocolate, this recipe will savor your cravings of chocolate in no time. Surprise your family and friends with this delicious sweet serving of Paleo Mexican Hot Chocolate Cupcakes.

Total Time Required
40 minutes

Nutritional Facts

Calories: 398.2
Cholesterol: 114.5mg
Carbohydrates: 39.6g
Protein: 8.9g
Fat: 25.9g

Ingredients for Cupcakes

Dark chocolate chips, ½ cup
Grass-fed unsalted butter, 1 cup
Pure vanilla extract, 1 tsp
Pure maple syrup, ½ cup
3 large eggs
Cocoa powder (unsweetened), 1/3 cup
Blanched almond flour, ¾ cups
Baking powder, 1 tsp
Sea salt, a pinch

Ingredients for Hot Chocolate Frosting

Dairy-free cream grass fed cheese,1 package
Grass-fed unsalted butter, ½ cup
Chili powder, 1 tsp
Ground cinnamon, ½ tsp
Pure vanilla extract, 1 tsp
Sea salt, ¼ tsp
Coconut sugar, (powdered)
Dark chocolate (unsweetened, melted), 3 oz

Preparation Method

Set the oven to preheat at 350°F. Prepare a cupcake pan with liners and set aside.

Prepare the batter for the cupcakes first. Take a large bowl (heat-resistant), add butter and chocolate and place over simmering skillet of water (make sure the bowl doesn't touch the bottom of the skillet). Stir to melt the ingredients and combine well. You can also combine butter and chocolate in a microwave if you prefer.

Stir in vanilla and maple syrup and combine well. Beat with an electric mixer until the ingredients are well incorporated and the mixture is smooth, for 2-3 minutes. Add eggs (one by one) and beat for another minute. Set aside.

In another bowl, sift together the dry ingredients including flour, baking powder, cocoa powder and salt. Combine with the wet mixture and blend to mix well.

Fill up the cupcake tray with the batter (2/3 of the full). Set to bake for 20 minutes until they are done and firm to touch.

Meanwhile, prepare the frosting. With an electric beater, beat together butter and cream grass fed cheese. Add cinnamon and chili powder and beat again to incorporate fully. Add coconut sugar, vanilla and salt and mix. Add in the melted chocolate and beat until the frosting is smooth.

When cupcakes are done, spread the frosting nicely and set to chill. Enjoy amazing, chocolaty flavors of this Mexican cupcake.

Frozen Chocolate Bananas
Serves 12

Enjoy the chocolate-dipped frozen bananas and relish the fruity Mexican dessert with friends and family. This Mexican-inspired sweet is simple to make and very delicious when served chilled directly from the freezer. Moreover, it requires very few, basic ingredients. Prepare now!

Total Time Required

40 minutes

Nutritional Facts

Calories: 212.4
Cholesterol: 24.3mg
Carbohydrates: 2.5g
Protein: 7.5g
Fat: 19.9g

Ingredients

Dark chocolate (finely chopped), 9 oz
Ground cinnamon, 1 tbsp
Olive oil, 1 tbsp
6 medium-sized bananas (halved crosswise)
Coconut flakes (toasted), 2 cups

Equipment Required

12 Pop sticks (wooden or craft)

Preparation Method

Combine oil, cinnamon and chocolate in a bowl and set in a microwave for a minute or two until the chocolate in melt and combine with the remaining ingredients.

Prepare a baking sheet and cover it with aluminum foil, silicone baking sheet or parchment paper. Insert pop sticks into the center of each piece of banana. Place the toasted coconut flakes in a plate.

When the chocolate mixture is prepared, pour in a shallow plate. Now pick up one banana with the stick and coat it with chocolate (one at a time). Once the entire banana is coated, roll it in the coconut flakes and place it on the baking sheet.

Repeat the process and coat all the bananas likewise. Place the baking dish in the freezer and let the bananas chill for at least 20 minutes.

Serve chilled and enjoy!

Mexican Cocktails – Everlasting Refreshment

Talking about the Tex-Mex menu, which is not complete without its special, refreshing cocktails.

Blend the refreshing Mexican flavors together and prepare the best drinks, you would love to serve. Check them out now!

Mystical Michelada

Serves 4

The cocktail native to the north of Mexico can now be prepared in your very own kitchen. The idea of a hot michelada comes from combining the flavors of beer and lime along with salt, chili and hot sauce. Try this unique Mexican spicy beer.

Total Time Required

5 minutes

Nutritional Facts

Calories: 116.4
Cholesterol: 0mg
Carbohydrates: 3.4g
Protein: 0g
Fat: 1.7g

Ingredients

Beer, 4 bottles of 12 oz
Sea salt, ¼ cup
Hot sauce (preferably Tabasco)
Chili powder, 3 tbsp
4 limes (slice into wedges)

Preparation Method

Mix together chili powder and salt in a plate. Rub lime on the rim of each glass or beer mug and place put the wet side on the plate to cover the rim with salt-chili.

Now squeeze lime juice into each of the four glasses or mugs. Put one wedge inside the glass. Add lots of ice into each glass or mug. Empty one bottle of beer into one glass. Drizzle hot sauce from top and serve the chilled, hot Michelada immediately.

Hot Margarita
Serves 1

Use this Mexican recipe to twist the class Margarita and make it hot and spicy. With an ounce of Grand Marnier, spicy tequila, sweet and sour mix and Serrano chilies for garnishing, you can turn up the heat instantly as you prepare this amazing and unique Mexican special margarita.

Total Time Required

5 minutes

Nutritional Facts

Calories: 82.5
Cholesterol: 0mg
Carbohydrates: 2.1g
Protein: 0g
Fat: 0g

Ingredients

Sauza Hornitos Tequila, 1 ½ oz
Ice
Spicy tequila, to taste
Grand marnier, 1 oz
Sweet and sour mix, 1 ¼ oz.
Paprika, to taste
Sea salt, to taste
Lime powder, to taste
Serrano Pepper, to taste

Preparation Method

In a pint glass, add ice and pour Sauza Hornitos tequila.

Add spicy tequila next according to the flavors you like. Add grand marnier and shake. Stir in sweet and sour mix and shake again to combine flavors.

Cover the glass rim with lime powder, salt and paprika. Use Serrano peppers for garnishing. Serve chilled.

Tequila Cocktail
Serves 2

The citrusy juices when combined with excellent quality tequila will give you a lifetime experience. Blend the pure Mexican flavors with honey and fresh mint and make this tequila cocktail refreshing for your taste buds. Serve chilled!

Total Time Required

5 minutes

Nutritional Facts

Calories: 111.7
Cholesterol: 0mg
Carbohydrates: 1.1g
Protein: 0g
Fat: 0g

Ingredients

Gold or white good quality tequila, 4 oz
Raw honey, 2 tsp
Juice of 1 orange
Juice of 1 lemon
Juice of 2 limes
Ice cubes
Mint leaves for garnish

Preparation Method

Add citrus juices, honey, and tequila in a cocktail shaker and shake until all the ingredients are well incorporated.

Add mint leaves and lots of ice in the shake and shake to make the mixture frothy. Pour into 2 glasses and garnish with mint. Serve chilled.

Agua Fresca

Serves 4

Agua Fresca, a Spanish word that stands for fresh water, is used for traditional fruity drinks prepared and served in Mexico. Feel free to use your favorite juicy cold fruits whichever you like and blend with ice, honey and fresh mind. For this recipe, we will use watermelon.

Total Time Required

10 minutes

Nutritional Facts

Calories: 92.1
Cholesterol: 0mg
Carbohydrates: 3.6g
Protein: 2.1g
Fat: 0g

Ingredients

1 small watermelon (diced and seeded)
Raw honey, ¼ cup
Fresh mint (chopped), a handful
Juice of 1 lime

Preparation Method

Add diced watermelon in a blender and pulse to puree. add water if required. Add ice and blend again. Strain watermelon puree through grass fed cheese-cloth if it is seedy or fibrous.

In a pitcher, add puree, along with some ice. Stir in chopped mint, lime juice and honey. Shake well and pour into four glasses. Enjoy fresh!

Get Started Now!

This lengthy Tex-Mex menu is all you need to prepare the best Mexican recipes at home without cheating on your Paleo diet.

The recipes are prepared with the best alternative ingredients to help you enjoy both taste and health at the same time. Enjoy the authentic, peppery taste of Mexican cuisine whether you are preparing sidelines, salsas, main course for breakfast, lunch or dinner, or savoring sweet Mexican dishes and cocktails.

Put your apron on and get started now!